Mastering Metabolism

"A Comprehensive Guide to Achieving Optimal Health and Fitness Through Nutrition"

By

Dr. Joshua M. Fields

Table of Contents

Table of Contents..3
Introduction 3
Understanding the Power of Your Metabolism 3
Chapter 1..3
Uncovering Metabolism 3
Chapter 2..3
Fundamentals of nutrition..3
i. What Macronutrients Do 3
ii. The Underrated Heroes of Micronutrients 3
iii. The Effects of Hydration on Metabolism...................................3
Chapter 3..3
The Science of Weight Loss 3
Chapter 4..3
Building a Metabolism-Boosting Diet..3
A Protein's Power 3
The Good, the Bad, and the Ugly of Fats 3
Energy and satiety from Carbohydrates 3
Chapter 5..3
Timing and Routine of Meals..3
In 3
i. How Important Breakfast Is 3
ii. Making Smart Snacks..3
iii. Is intermittent fasting a good or bad thing?..............................3
Chapter 6..3
Exercise's Function 3
In 3
i. Metabolic Rate and Exercise 3
ii. Cardio, strength, and flexibility combined 3
iii. Exercise to Manage Weight 3
Chapter 7..3
Aging and Metabolism 3
The crucial relationship between metabolism and aging is discussed
in 3
i. How Aging Affects Metabolism 3

ii. Optimal Nutrition for Healthy Aging 3
iii. Exercise During Your Golden Years 3
Chapter 8...3
Special Diets and Metabolism 3
investigates the realm of dietary constraints and how they effect
metabolism. This chapter includes three main parts: 3
i. Various Popular Diets...3
Exploring Keto, Paleo, Vegan, and More...................................3
ii. Dietary Restriction's Effect on Metabolism 3
iii. Finding the Diet that Is Right for Me.................................3
Chapter 9...3
Prevention of Disease and Metabolism 3
Chronic Diseases and Metabolism 3
Nutritional Strategies to Lower Disease Risk............................3
Supplements' Function...3
Chapter 10..3
Beyond Weight: Lifelong Wellness 3
i. Nutritional Care for Mental Health 3
ii. Rest and Recuperation..3
iii. Stress and hormone balance 3
Chapter 11..3
Ethical Eating and Sustainability...3
In 3
i. The Effects of Food Choices on the Environment 3
ii. Ethical Issues Regarding Nutrition.....................................3
iii. Make Informed Decisions 3
The Verdict: Control Your Metabolism for Lifelong Health 3
Your Metabolic Journey in Review 3
Taking Initiative for Lifelong Wellness 3
Adopting a Lifestyle Driven by Metabolism..............................3
Chapter 12..3
Chapter 14..3
Reflecting on Your Metabolic Journey: 3
3.)Hydration Habits: 3
Mastering Metabolism..1

Introduction

Understanding the Power of Your Metabolism

In the first chapter of "Mastering Metabolism," we go on a quest to understand the fundamental importance of your metabolism—a dynamic force that plays a critical role in determining your health, energy, and longevity. This introduction lays the foundation for the transforming knowledge that follows in the book, examining three essential aspects:

Why Your Metabolism Matters

Your metabolism isn't simply a biological process; it's the quiet engine pushing your body's operations. This section looks into the sheer importance of metabolism, demonstrating how it regulates energy expenditure, manages weight, and promotes general well-being. By understanding why your metabolism matters, you'll acquire important insights into its ability to alter your life.

The Connection Between Metabolism and Health

This chapter delves beneath the surface and plunges into the complicated link

between metabolism and health. It unravels how metabolism effects everything from illness prevention to mental well-being, delivering a deep awareness for the immense control your metabolism exerts over your body. It's a relationship that, if comprehended, will enable you to make educated decisions and take responsibility for your health path.
Setting the Stage for Lifelong Wellness
As we complete the introduction, we establish a goal for the future—one of permanent wellbeing. You'll discover how knowing and managing your metabolism might

be the key to unlocking a lifetime of vitality, energy, and good health. By setting this stage for lifetime wellbeing, you'll be encouraged to begin on a path of self-discovery and empowerment, equipped with the information and resources required to have a lasting good influence on your life. This introduction is the first step in a revolutionary adventure into the realm of metabolism, and it's a trip that promises to equip you with the information and insights essential to improve your health and well-being. As you explore further into the pages that follow, you'll find the remarkable power of your metabolism to change your future and increase your quality of life.

Chapter 1

Uncovering Metabolism

In the first chapter of "Mastering Metabolism," we begin out on a fascinating adventure to solve the metabolic problems. This chapter, which comprises three important components, provides the foundation of our examination of metabolic health.

Getting the Metabolism in Order

The process of metabolism is generally regarded to be mysterious and complex. But in this part, we lift the veil of mystery and make the inner workings of metabolism clear to everyone. You'll find a new respect for how your body's metabolism operates via simple explanations and realistic examples. We empower you to confront this key part of your physiology with confidence and clarity by demystifying metabolism.

Both nourishment and vitality

All biological operations are pushed by energy, and metabolism is the mechanism that provides that energy. We dive into the delicate link between metabolism and energy production in this portion of the chapter. You'll discover how successfully your body turns the food you consume into the energy required to power your everyday activities. To increase your energy levels and employ the utmost potential of your metabolism, it is vital to grasp this relationship. Either a quick or a sluggish metabolism—which is preferable?

The notion of metabolism is not universal. The interesting issue of metabolic variability—the concept that humans may have varying rates of metabolism—is discussed in this section. We break down the components that determine metabolism speed and give advice on how to leverage your individual metabolic profile to reach your fitness and health goals. You'll be better equipped to adjust your food and lifestyle choices for the greatest outcomes if you are aware of the tiny variances between different metabolic types.

Metabolism revealing Your doorway into the inner workings of one of the most fundamental biological processes is "Metabolism Unveiled". You'll start to grasp the vast power you hold as we uncover the secrets of metabolism, analyze its role in the creation of energy, and explore the diversity of metabolic types. This chapter establishes the basis for your quest for metabolic mastery by giving you the knowledge essential to make informed choices and start along the path to long-term wellbeing.

Chapter 2

Fundamentals of nutrition

In "Chapter 2: Nutrition Fundamentals" of "Mastering

Metabolism," we dig deeply into the fundamentals of nutrition to give you a rock-solid knowledge of how your food selections affect your metabolism and overall health. *This chapter is broken into three major sections:*

i. What Macronutrients Do

Proteins repair and build tissues, carbohydrates supply energy, and fats support important processes; these are the macronutrients at the heart of nutrition. In this part, we uncover the power of macronutrients, clarifying their functions in the body. Equipped with this information, you'll be able to build a well-balanced diet that properly feeds your metabolism.

ii. The Underrated Heroes of Micronutrients

We study how micronutrients are involved in energy generation, immunological function, and general health. Understanding the relevance of micronutrients offers you the knowledge required to ensure your diet is nutritionally sufficient. While macronutrients receive all the attention, micronutrients are the hidden heroes of nutrition. These vitamins and minerals are needed for several biochemical processes in your body, and this section emphasizes their crucial functions.

iii. The Effects of Hydration on Metabolism

The tremendous influence of water on metabolism is discussed in this portion of the chapter. You'll discover how water is involved in practically every biological activity, from digestion to temperature control. Discover the consequences of dehydration and discover practical ideas for maintaining adequate water levels to support your metabolic health. Nutrition Fundamentals serves as the cornerstone of your quest to metabolic mastery. By knowing the responsibilities of macronutrients and micronutrients, as well as respecting the necessity of water, you'll be well-prepared to make smart dictary decisions. This understanding is the key to optimizing your metabolism, ensuring that you nourish your body in a manner that promotes energy, vitality, and long-term well-being.

Chapter 3

The Science of Weight Loss

In "Chapter 3: The Science of Weight Loss" of "Mastering Metabolism," we dig deeper into the complicated systems regulating weight management and study the science behind it. Calories In, Calories Out: An Easy Method You'll learn how to balance your energy intake with expenditure, providing you a good basis for your weight control journey. Weight control frequently looks difficult, but at its foundation, it's a question of calories in against calories out. In this part, we simplify the weight loss equation, making it accessible and simple to grasp.

Regulation of Metabolism and Weight Understanding this link is vital for successful and sustained weight control since metabolism plays a fundamental role in weight regulation. You'll discover how your metabolism effects the storage and burning of calories, providing light on why some individuals may find it easier to lose weight than others.

Common Myths Dispelled About Weight Loss

With this information, you'll be more able to make educated choices on your weight reduction journey and avoid the traps that commonly inhibit success. The weight loss landscape is plagued with myths and misunderstandings. In this section, we refute some of the most prominent weight reduction misconceptions, separating reality from fiction.

Chapter 4

Building a Metabolism-Boosting Diet

Building a metabolism-boosting diet is described in "Chapter 4: Harnessing Your Metabolism to Achieve Your Health and Fitness Goals," which is a vital step in leveraging your metabolism to your advantage.
Making Your Perfect Plate
In this part, you'll learn the foundations of portion management and nutritional distribution, ensuring that your meals are adjusted to support

your metabolic health.
Creating a balanced and
metabolism-friendly diet
starts with understanding
how to design the ideal
plate.

A Protein's Power

This discover how
protein assists in muscle
maintenance, maintains
satiety, and contributes
to a well-rounded diet as
this portion of the
chapter discusses
protein's importance.
You'll acquire insights
on the greatest sources of
protein and how to
include them into your
meals.

The Good, the Bad, and the Ugly of Fats

We analyze the distinctions between good and poor fats, emphasizing their significance in metabolic health, and demystify the challenging issue of fats in nutrition in this part. By the finish, you'll have a complete knowledge of how to pick healthy fats that boost your metabolism.

Energy and satiety from Carbohydrates

In this portion of the chapter, we investigate the function that carbohydrates play in

supporting your
metabolism. You'll learn
how to pick the correct
carbs for lasting energy
and satiety while also
managing blood sugar
levels.
By learning the science
of weight reduction and
the foundations of
nutrition, you'll be well-
prepared to make smart
nutritional choices and
achieve sustained
success in your health
and fitness journey.

Chapter 5

Timing and Routine of Meals

In "Chapter 5, Meal Timing and Frequency" of "Mastering Metabolism," we study the intricate link between the time and frequency of your meals and their influence on your metabolic health. *This chapter is broken into three essential sections:*

i. How Important Breakfast Is

Breakfast is generally referred to be the most essential meal of the day, but why? In this part, we discuss the science underlying breakfast's relevance and its impact on metabolism and overall health. You'll discover how beginning your day with a healthy breakfast may enhance your metabolism.

ii. Making Smart Snacks

Snacking is a frequent behavior, but not all snacks are made equal. This portion of the chapter addresses the art of snacking sensibly. You'll discover how to pick nutrient-rich and metabolism-friendly snacks that deliver continuous energy throughout the day, without the dreaded energy collapses.

iii. Is intermittent fasting a good or bad thing?

This section explores the idea of intermittent fasting, shedding light on its potential advantages and disadvantages, so by the time you're done, you'll have a thorough understanding of whether intermittent fasting is right for you and whether it will help you achieve your goals and lead a fulfilling lifestyle.

Chapter 6

Exercise's Function

In "Chapter 6, The Role of Exercise," we look into the symbiotic link between physical activity and metabolism. *This chapter addresses three key components:*

i. Metabolic Rate and Exercise

This section covers the dynamic link between metabolism and exercise and how various forms of physical activity, from cardio to strength

training, impact your
metabolic rate and
overall health. Physical
exercise is a stimulant
for metabolic processes.

ii. Cardio, strength, and flexibility combined

This portion of the
chapter talks you
through the benefits of
mixing cardio, weight
training, and flexibility
exercises to help you
design a holistic fitness
routine that supports
your metabolic
objectives and enhances
your overall well-being.

iii. Exercise to Manage Weight

This section analyzes the science behind doing exercise for weight control, putting light on the most effective techniques for accomplishing your desired aims. Weight management is a common fitness goal, and exercise plays a significant element in obtaining and maintaining a healthy weight.
Making informed judgments in these areas will help you to better harness the power of your metabolism and start on a road to long-

term fitness and vitality. These chapters provide you a full grasp of how meal time, frequency, and activity effect your metabolism and general health.

Chapter 7

Aging and Metabolism

The crucial relationship between metabolism and aging is discussed in "Chapter 7: Metabolism and Aging" of "Mastering Metabolism," *which is divided down into three key sections:*

i. How Aging Affects Metabolism

Understanding these changes is vital to changing your lifestyle and nutritional choices to promote healthy aging.

As we become older, our
metabolism alters
substantially. In this part,
we investigate these
alterations, from a drop
in metabolic rate to
changes in dietary needs.

ii. Optimal Nutrition for Healthy Aging

This portion of the
chapter gives insights
into dietary practices
customized to the
requirements of older
persons. You'll discover
how to modify your diet
to handle age-related
difficulties, such as
retaining muscle mass,
managing chronic
illnesses, and supporting
cognitive health.
Nutrition is a great tool

for maintaining general
health and well-being as
we age.

iii. Exercise During Your Golden Years

We study how regular exercise might reduce the consequences of aging on metabolism, mobility, and vitality. You'll learn practical strategies for integrating physical exercise into your everyday routine, ensuring that you stay active and bright as you age. In this part, we underline the necessity of remaining active in your senior years.

Chapter 8

Special Diets and Metabolism

investigates the realm of dietary constraints and how they effect metabolism. *This chapter includes three main parts:*

i. Various Popular Diets

Exploring Keto, Paleo, Vegan, and More

You'll have a broad grasp of diverse nutritional approaches at the conclusion of this part, which takes you on a trip to study well-known diets including keto, paleo, and veganism. We look at the basic concepts of these diets, their possible benefits, and their impact on metabolism.

ii. Dietary Restriction's Effect on Metabolism

You'll get insights into the possible advantages and problems connected with dietary limitations and how they may correspond with your health and lifestyle objectives in this portion of the chapter, where we dig into the ways that diets like keto and veganism might alter metabolic processes.

iii. Finding the Diet that Is Right for Me

We give practical recommendations for analyzing your objectives, interests, and dietary needs to make educated choices about the best suited diet for your metabolic health and overall well-being. By adopting dietary and lifestyle recommendations targeted to your unique requirements, you'll be better equipped to manage the aging process and make choices that promote your health and vitality. These chapters provide you a complete grasp of

how metabolism varies
with age and how dietary
choices, including
special diets, might
effect your metabolic
health.

Chapter 9

Prevention of Disease
and Metabolism

In "Chapter 9:
Metabolism and Disease
Prevention" of
"Mastering Metabolism,"
we look into the essential
role metabolism plays in
safeguarding your health
against chronic illnesses.

Chronic Diseases and Metabolism

Understanding the complicated links between metabolism and illnesses like diabetes, heart disease, and cancer can help you to take preventive strategies to minimize your disease risk. In this part, we study the subtle relationships between metabolism and illnesses including diabetes, heart disease, and cancer.

Nutritional Strategies to Lower Disease Risk

You'll learn about the foods and nutrients that play a critical role in disease prevention and gain practical guidance on integrating them into your regular meals in this portion of the chapter, which gives insights into how you may utilize your diet to lower illness risk.

Supplements' Function

This section covers the function of supplements in maintaining metabolic health and decreasing disease risk; you'll get insights into when and how to utilize supplements effectively and safely as part of your overall wellness plan. While a well-balanced diet is the cornerstone of health, supplements may also play a role in illness prevention.

Chapter 10

Beyond Weight: Lifelong Wellness

Beyond Weight: Lifelong Wellness" gives a comprehensive approach to wellness *and covers three crucial elements:*

i. Nutritional Care for Mental Health

You'll learn about the foods and dietary patterns that boost emotional balance, cognitive function, and mental resilience in this portion, which analyzes how nutrition may encourage your mental well-being.

ii. Rest and Recuperation

This portion of the chapter looks into the science of sleep and its implications on metabolism and overall health. You'll discover practical tactics for improving your sleep and recovery patterns, ensuring that you wake up feeling refreshed and ready to tackle each day.

This section covers approaches to reduce stress and maintain hormonal balance via food and lifestyle choices. You'll discover ways for minimizing stress and improving hormonal equilibrium to sustain lifetime wellbeing. Stress and hormonal imbalances may damage metabolic health and well-being. By addressing both physical and mental aspects of well-being, you'll be better equipped to lead a fulfilling, healthy, and balanced life.These chapters provide you with a comprehensive understanding of how metabolism influences the development and prevention of chronic diseases and how you can use nutrition, supplements, and lifestyle choices to reduce disease risk and promote lifelong wellness.

Chapter 11

Ethical Eating and Sustainability

In "Chapter 11: Sustainability and Ethical Eating" of "Mastering Metabolism," we

transfer our focus to the larger effect of our food choices on the environment and ethical nutrition problems. *This chapter is broken into three essential sections:*

i. The Effects of Food Choices on the Environment

Our dietary choices have a big influence on the environment, and in this part, we investigate the implications of different diets and food production systems. You'll discover how your eating choices may encourage sustainability and lower your ecological impact.

ii. Ethical Issues Regarding Nutrition

This portion of the chapter looks into themes including animal welfare, fair trading, and food justice. By looking at these ethical elements of nutrition, you'll be ready to make choices that are compatible with your values and beliefs. Ethical issues in diet extend beyond human health to cover wider ethical and moral concepts.

iii. Make Informed Decisions

You'll learn about certifications, labels, and

tools that may help you make choices that are not only healthy for you but also ethical and sustainable for the world. Making educated selections in a world full with food alternatives is vital. This section includes tips on how to negotiate ethical and sustainable eating.

The Verdict: Control Your Metabolism for Lifelong Health

In the last chapter of "Mastering Metabolism," we take a look back at your metabolic journey and provide you solid advice for preserving heath throughout your life.

You've been on a transformative adventure through the realm of metabolism, and in this portion, we encourage you to take a time to stop and evaluate what you've learned. You'll have a greater knowledge of the power of your metabolism and how it influences every part of your life.

Taking Initiative for Lifelong Wellness

From diet and exercise to sleep and stress management, you'll gain practical tips for achieving lifetime wellbeing. This section gives concrete, attainable measures that you may adopt into your everyday life to maintain and strengthen your metabolic health.

Adopting a Lifestyle Driven by Metabolism

You'll feel more empowered and inspired to live a metabolism-driven lifestyle as you finish your journey through "Mastering Metabolism," knowing that you are in charge of your metabolic health and overall well-being. In the last chapter, you'll reflect on your metabolic journey and get specific steps for adopting a lifetime commitment to health and wellbeing, guided by the information and insights learned throughout the book. These chapters give a complete overview of the environmental, ethical, and sustainability elements of nutrition, allowing you to make decisions that line with your beliefs and have a beneficial influence on the earth.

Chapter 12

Appendix A: Sample Meal Plans and Recipes

In this appendix, we present a practical guide to implementing the principles of metabolism-boosting nutrition with a diverse range of sample meal plans and mouth watering recipes. Whether you're aiming for weight loss, muscle gain, improved energy, or balanced nutrition, we've curated meal ideas that cater to your specific health and fitness goals.

Meal Ideas for Different Goals:

Tailoring nutrition to individual goals is crucial. We provide detailed sample meal plans that consider various objectives: **Weight Loss:** Discover nutrient-dense, low-calorie meals that support weight loss without compromising on taste or satisfaction.

Muscle Gain: Explore protein-rich meals designed to fuel muscle growth, including a balance of carbohydrates and healthy fats to support energy and recovery.

Improved Energy: Unlock the potential of meals that focus on sustained energy release, incorporating complex carbohydrates and nutrient-dense foods to keep you energized throughout the day.

Balanced Nutrition: Delve into well-rounded meal plans that provide a mix of macronutrients and micronutrients, promoting overall health and vitality.

Each meal plan comes with detailed recipes, portion sizes, and nutritional information, ensuring that readers can easily incorporate these plans into their daily lives.

Delicious and Nutrient-Packed Recipes:

Elevate your culinary experience with our collection of recipes designed to align with the principles of metabolism-boosting nutrition. Each recipe is crafted to not only tantalize your taste buds but also deliver essential nutrients that support your metabolic health:

Breakfast Delights: From energizing smoothie bowls to protein-packed omelets, kickstart your day with recipes that set a positive tone for metabolic activity.

Lunchtime Favorites: Explore satisfying and nutritious lunch options, ranging from vibrant salads to hearty soups, ensuring you stay fueled and focused.

Dinner Creations: End your day with a variety of flavorful dinner recipes, including lean proteins, healthy fats, and wholesome carbohydrates to support recovery and metabolic function.

Snacks and Desserts: Indulge guilt-free with nutrient-packed snacks and desserts that satisfy your cravings while contributing to your overall health.

Chapter 14

Conclusion
Mastering Your Metabolism for a Lifetime of Health

Reflecting on Your Metabolic Journey:

Take a moment to reflect on the insights gained throughout your metabolic journey. Consider the knowledge acquired about your body, nutrition, and the profound connection between metabolism and overall health. Recognize the positive changes, both big and small, and celebrate the progress made on your path to optimal well-being.

Actionable Steps for Lifelong Wellness:

To ensure the journey doesn't end with the last page, we provide concrete and actionable steps for readers to incorporate into their daily lives:

1.)Mindful Eating Practices: Cultivate awareness around mealtime, savoring each bite, and paying attention to hunger and fullness cues.

2.)Regular Physical Activity: Establish a consistent exercise

routine that includes a
mix of cardiovascular,
strength, and flexibility
exercises tailored to
individual preferences
and fitness levels.

3.)Hydration Habits:

Prioritize proper
hydration by
incorporating water-rich
foods and maintaining a
regular water intake
routine throughout the
day.

4.)Balanced Nutrition:

Strive for a
balanced diet that includes
a variety of nutrient-dense
foods, promoting overall
health and supporting
metabolic function.

5.) Prioritize sufficient and restful

sleep,
recognizing its impact on

metabolism, cognitive
function, and overall
well-being.

**6.)*Stress Management
Techniques:*** Adopt stress-
reducing practices such as
meditation, deep breathing
exercises, or engaging in
hobbies to promote a
balanced and resilient
mindset.

7.)*Lifelong Learning:*
Stay informed about
evolving nutritional
science, wellness
practices, and sustainable
living, fostering a mindset
of continuous
improvement.

Embracing a Metabolism-Driven Lifestyle:

Inspire readers to go
beyond short-term goals
and embrace a lifestyle
centered around

understanding and optimizing their metabolism. Encourage them to view nutrition not as a restrictive regimen but as a dynamic, lifelong journey. By embracing a metabolism-driven lifestyle, individuals can foster a profound connection with their bodies, making informed choices that contribute to sustained health, vitality, and longevity.